This diet and exercise journal belongs to …

....

....

....

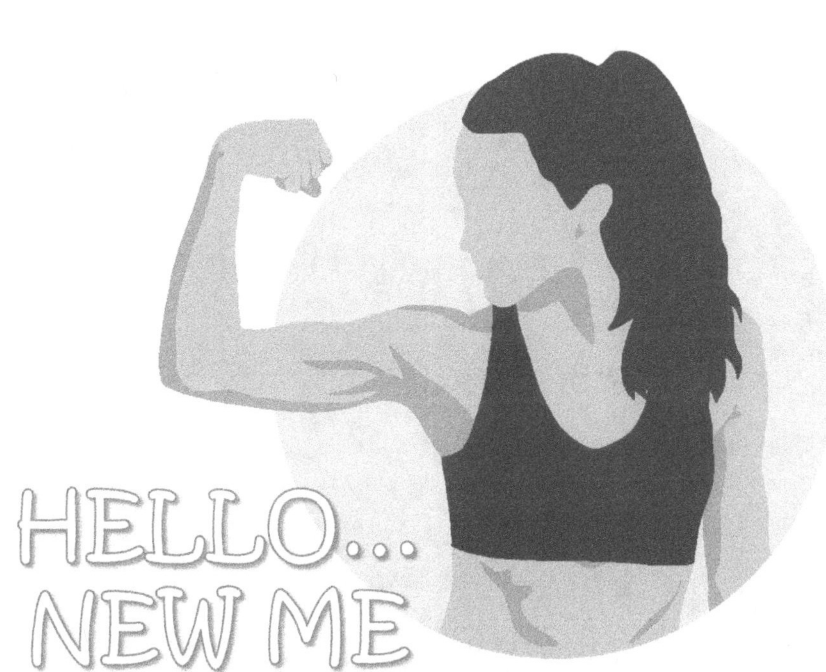

15 TIPS
To Get You Started

1. Drink enough water to keep you hydrated.
2. Eat green and leafy kind vegetables and the orange and red ones.
3. Enjoy some fruit everyday too
4. Avoid processed food and quickly digested carbs.
5. Eat more complex carbs or whole grains, lean proteins, fish, eggs, fat-free daily and lean meat.
6. MOVE, MOVE, and MOVE some more!
7. Stretch daily to increase flexibility
8. Chew your food at least 20 to 30 times before you swallow it.
9. Think before putting something into your mount.
10. Try yoga or meditation.
11. Go to bed earlier.
12. Keep tracking on your progress.
13. Enjoy your progress even it's small.
14. Do not compare yourself to others.
15. Do not give up. If you want to give up remember why you started.

Cross a big "X" over each day you completed your daily goals.

Week 1	1	2	3	4	5	6	7
Week 2	8	9	10	11	12	13	14
Week 3	15	16	17	18	19	20	21
Week 4	22	23	24	25	26	27	28
Week 5	29	30	31	32	33	34	35
Week 6	36	37	38	39	40	41	42
Week 7	42	44	45	46	47	48	49
Week 8	50	51	53	53	54	55	56
Week 9	57	58	59	60	61	62	63
Week 10	64	65	66	67	68	69	70
Week 11	71	72	73	74	75	76	77
Week 12	78	79	80	81	82	83	84
Week 13	85	86	87	88	89	90	

30 days — Break Unhealthy Habits

60 days — Celebrate Your Progress

90 days — Enjoy Your Success

Consistency is a Magic Wand!

BODY PROGRAM

BEFORE

DATE ___________

NECK ___________
ARM ___________
CHEST ___________
WAIST ___________
HIP ___________
THIGH ___________
CALF ___________
BMI ___________

WEIGHT

AFTER

DATE ___________

NECK ___________
ARM ___________
CHEST ___________
WAIST ___________
HIP ___________
THIGH ___________
CALF ___________
BMI ___________

WEIGHT

PROGRESS TRACKER

	W1	W2	W3	W4	W5	W6	W7	W8	W9	W10	W11	W12	W13
NECK													
BICEP													
CHEST													
WAIST													
HIP													
THIGH													
CALF													
BMI													
WEIGHT													

WHERE DO I WANT TO BE?

It's important to set goals for a week that are specific and measurable. Revisit them often to stay on track.

- [ ] **GOAL#1** ____
  Deadline ___________ Plan ___________________________

- [ ] **GOAL#2** ____
  Deadline ___________ Plan ___________________________

- [ ] **GOAL#3** ____
  Deadline ___________ Plan ___________________________

- [ ] **GOAL#4** ____
  Deadline ___________ Plan ___________________________

- [ ] **GOAL#5** ____
  Deadline ___________ Plan ___________________________

- [ ] **GOAL#6** ____
  Deadline ___________ Plan ___________________________

- [ ] **GOAL#7** ____
  Deadline ___________ Plan ___________________________

- [ ] **GOAL#8** ____
  Deadline ___________ Plan ___________________________

- [ ] **GOAL#9** ____
  Deadline ___________ Plan ___________________________

- [ ] **GOAL#10** ____
  Deadline ___________ Plan ___________________________

- [ ] **GOAL#11** ____
  Deadline ___________ Plan ___________________________

- [ ] **GOAL#12** ____
  Deadline ___________ Plan ___________________________

- [ ] **GOAL#13** ____
  Deadline ___________ Plan ___________________________

MY IDEAL LIFE

LIFE GOALS	HEALTH GOALS

COMMITMENT TO MYSELF • PLAN FOR ACTIONS

You are what you believe to be true.

I am healthy and full of energy.

I am stronger than any excuse.

I am in control of my eating habits.

I am losing weight.

I am unstoppable.

M T W T F S S   MOOD     **DAY** | 1

DATE ....

TODAY'S COMMITMENTS

____

____

TODAY MEALS	BREAKFAST	LUNCH	DINNER	SNACKS
	Calories:	Calories:	Calories:	Calories:

FATS	CARBS	PROTEINS	OTHERS

WATER ⎕ ⎕ ⎕ ⎕ ⎕ ⎕ ⎕ ⎕   SLEEP   WEIGHT

WORKOUT ACTIVITIES / EXERCISES	SET / REPS / DISTANCE	CALORIES BURNED	TIME SPENT

NOTES/TODAY'S ACHIEVEMENT	WHAT WILL DO BETTER TOMORROW

M T W T F S S   MOOD   **DAY** | 2

DATE ....

TODAY'S COMMITMENTS

____

____

____

<table>
<tr><td rowspan="2">TODAY MEALS</td><td>BREAKFAST</td><td>LUNCH</td><td>DINNER</td><td>SNACKS</td></tr>
<tr><td>Calories:</td><td>Calories:</td><td>Calories:</td><td>Calories:</td></tr>
</table>

FATS	CARBS	PROTEINS	OTHERS

WATER ▢▢▢▢▢▢▢▢   ⏰ SLEEP   WEIGHT

WORKOUT ACTIVITIES / EXERCISES	SET / REPS / DISTANCE	CALORIES BURNED	TIME SPENT

NOTES/TODAY'S ACHIEVEMENT	WHAT WILL DO BETTER TOMORROW

M T W T F S S MOOD   **DAY** | 3 |

DATE ....

TODAY'S COMMITMENTS

<table>
<tr><td rowspan="7">TODAY MEALS</td><td>BREAKFAST</td><td>LUNCH</td><td>DINNER</td><td>SNACKS</td></tr>
<tr><td></td><td></td><td></td><td></td></tr>
<tr><td></td><td></td><td></td><td></td></tr>
<tr><td></td><td></td><td></td><td></td></tr>
<tr><td></td><td></td><td></td><td></td></tr>
<tr><td></td><td></td><td></td><td></td></tr>
<tr><td>Calories:</td><td>Calories:</td><td>Calories:</td><td>Calories:</td></tr>
</table>

FATS	CARBS	PROTEINS	OTHERS

WATER ☐ ☐ ☐ ☐ ☐ ☐ ☐ ☐   SLEEP   WEIGHT

WORKOUT ACTIVITIES / EXERCISES	SET / REPS / DISTANCE	CALORIES BURNED	TIME SPENT

NOTES/TODAY'S ACHIEVEMENT	WHAT WILL DO BETTER TOMORROW

M T W T F S S   MOOD  

DATE ....

DAY | 4

TODAY'S COMMITMENTS

TODAY MEALS	BREAKFAST	LUNCH	DINNER	SNACKS
	Calories:	Calories:	Calories:	Calories:

FATS	CARBS	PROTEINS	OTHERS

WATER   SLEEP   WEIGHT

WORKOUT ACTIVITIES / EXERCISES	SET / REPS / DISTANCE	CALORIES BURNED	TIME SPENT

NOTES/TODAY'S ACHIEVEMENT	WHAT WILL DO BETTER TOMORROW

M T W T F S S   MOOD 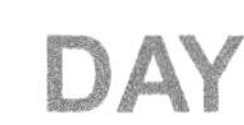 **DAY** | 5

DATE ....

TODAY'S COMMITMENTS

TODAY MEALS	BREAKFAST	LUNCH	DINNER	SNACKS
	Calories:	Calories:	Calories:	Calories:

FATS	CARBS	PROTEINS	OTHERS

WATER ⬚ ⬚ ⬚ ⬚ ⬚ ⬚ ⬚ ⬚   SLEEP   WEIGHT

WORKOUT ACTIVITIES / EXERCISES	SET / REPS / DISTANCE	CALORIES BURNED	TIME SPENT

NOTES/TODAY'S ACHIEVEMENT	WHAT WILL DO BETTER TOMORROW

M T W T F S S   MOOD 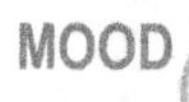   

DAY 6

DATE ....

TODAY'S COMMITMENTS

____

____

TODAY MEALS	BREAKFAST	LUNCH	DINNER	SNACKS
	Calories:	Calories:	Calories:	Calories:

FATS	CARBS	PROTEINS	OTHERS

WATER 🥤🥤🥤🥤🥤🥤🥤🥤   ⏰ SLEEP   WEIGHT

WORKOUT ACTIVITIES / EXERCISES	SET / REPS / DISTANCE	CALORIES BURNED	TIME SPENT

NOTES/TODAY'S ACHIEVEMENT	WHAT WILL DO BETTER TOMORROW

M T W T F S S   MOOD 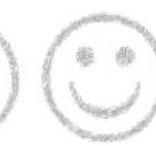 

DAY 7

DATE ....

TODAY'S COMMITMENTS

____

____

TODAY MEALS	BREAKFAST	LUNCH	DINNER	SNACKS
	Calories:	Calories:	Calories:	Calories:

FATS	CARBS	PROTEINS	OTHERS

WATER	SLEEP	WEIGHT

WORKOUT ACTIVITIES / EXERCISES	SET / REPS / DISTANCE	CALORIES BURNED	TIME SPENT

NOTES/TODAY'S ACHIEVEMENT	WHAT WILL DO BETTER TOMORROW

DATE ....

DAY | 8

TODAY'S COMMITMENTS

___

TODAY MEALS	BREAKFAST	LUNCH	DINNER	SNACKS
	Calories:	Calories:	Calories:	Calories:

FATS	CARBS	PROTEINS	OTHERS

WATER ⬜⬜⬜⬜⬜⬜⬜⬜   SLEEP   WEIGHT

WORKOUT ACTIVITIES / EXERCISES	SET / REPS / DISTANCE	CALORIES BURNED	TIME SPENT

NOTES/TODAY'S ACHIEVEMENT	WHAT WILL DO BETTER TOMORROW

M T W T F S S MOOD   DAY | 9

DATE ....

TODAY'S COMMITMENTS

TODAY MEALS	BREAKFAST	LUNCH	DINNER	SNACKS
	Calories:	Calories:	Calories:	Calories:

FATS	CARBS	PROTEINS	OTHERS

WATER 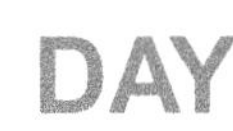   SLEEP   WEIGHT

WORKOUT ACTIVITIES / EXERCISES	SET / REPS / DISTANCE	CALORIES BURNED	TIME SPENT

NOTES/TODAY'S ACHIEVEMENT	WHAT WILL DO BETTER TOMORROW

M T W T F S S MOOD   **DAY 10**

DATE ....

TODAY'S COMMITMENTS

<table>
<tr><td rowspan="2">TODAY MEALS</td><td>BREAKFAST</td><td>LUNCH</td><td>DINNER</td><td>SNACKS</td></tr>
<tr><td>Calories:</td><td>Calories:</td><td>Calories:</td><td>Calories:</td></tr>
</table>

FATS	CARBS	PROTEINS	OTHERS

WATER SLEEP WEIGHT

WORKOUT ACTIVITIES / EXERCISES	SET / REPS / DISTANCE	CALORIES BURNED	TIME SPENT

NOTES/TODAY'S ACHIEVEMENT	WHAT WILL DO BETTER TOMORROW

M T W T F S S   MOOD 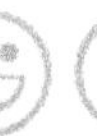 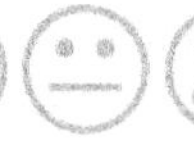 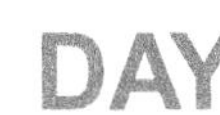   **DAY** 11

DATE ....

TODAY'S COMMITMENTS

____

____

<table>
<tr><td rowspan="2">TODAY MEALS</td><td>BREAKFAST</td><td>LUNCH</td><td>DINNER</td><td>SNACKS</td></tr>
<tr><td>Calories:</td><td>Calories:</td><td>Calories:</td><td>Calories:</td></tr>
</table>

FATS	CARBS	PROTEINS	OTHERS

WATER ☐ ☐ ☐ ☐ ☐ ☐ ☐ ☐   SLEEP   WEIGHT

WORKOUT ACTIVITIES / EXERCISES	SET / REPS / DISTANCE	CALORIES BURNED	TIME SPENT

NOTES/TODAY'S ACHIEVEMENT	WHAT WILL DO BETTER TOMORROW

M T W T F S S   MOOD   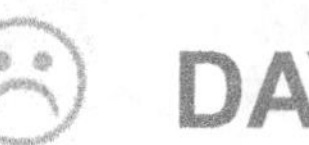   **DAY** | 12

DATE ....

TODAY'S COMMITMENTS

<table>
<tr><th rowspan="7">TODAY MEALS</th><th>BREAKFAST</th><th>LUNCH</th><th>DINNER</th><th>SNACKS</th></tr>
<tr><td></td><td></td><td></td><td></td></tr>
<tr><td></td><td></td><td></td><td></td></tr>
<tr><td></td><td></td><td></td><td></td></tr>
<tr><td></td><td></td><td></td><td></td></tr>
<tr><td></td><td></td><td></td><td></td></tr>
<tr><td>Calories:</td><td>Calories:</td><td>Calories:</td><td>Calories:</td></tr>
</table>

FATS	CARBS	PROTEINS	OTHERS

WATER ☐ ☐ ☐ ☐ ☐ ☐ ☐ ☐   SLEEP   WEIGHT

WORKOUT ACTIVITIES / EXERCISES	SET / REPS / DISTANCE	CALORIES BURNED	TIME SPENT

NOTES/TODAY'S ACHIEVEMENT	WHAT WILL DO BETTER TOMORROW

M T W T F S S   MOOD   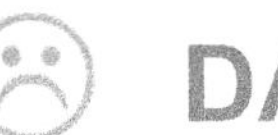   **DAY** | 13

DATE ....

TODAY'S COMMITMENTS

___

<table>
<tr><td rowspan="2">TODAY MEALS</td><td>BREAKFAST</td><td>LUNCH</td><td>DINNER</td><td>SNACKS</td></tr>
<tr><td>Calories:</td><td>Calories:</td><td>Calories:</td><td>Calories:</td></tr>
</table>

FATS	CARBS	PROTEINS	OTHERS

WATER □ □ □ □ □ □ □ □   SLEEP   WEIGHT

WORKOUT ACTIVITIES / EXERCISES	SET / REPS / DISTANCE	CALORIES BURNED	TIME SPENT

NOTES/TODAY'S ACHIEVEMENT	WHAT WILL DO BETTER TOMORROW

M T W T F S S   MOOD 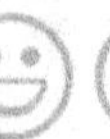     DAY 14

DATE ....

TODAY'S COMMITMENTS

____

____

TODAY MEALS	BREAKFAST	LUNCH	DINNER	SNACKS
	Calories:	Calories:	Calories:	Calories:

FATS	CARBS	PROTEINS	OTHERS

WATER 🥛🥛🥛🥛🥛🥛🥛🥛   ⏰ SLEEP   WEIGHT

WORKOUT ACTIVITIES / EXERCISES	SET / REPS / DISTANCE	CALORIES BURNED	TIME SPENT

NOTES/TODAY'S ACHIEVEMENT	WHAT WILL DO BETTER TOMORROW

M T W T F S S   MOOD   **DAY** 15

DATE ....

TODAY'S COMMITMENTS

<table>
<tr><td rowspan="6">TODAY MEALS</td><td>BREAKFAST</td><td>LUNCH</td><td>DINNER</td><td>SNACKS</td></tr>
<tr><td></td><td></td><td></td><td></td></tr>
<tr><td>Calories:</td><td>Calories:</td><td>Calories:</td><td>Calories:</td></tr>
</table>

FATS	CARBS	PROTEINS	OTHERS

WATER 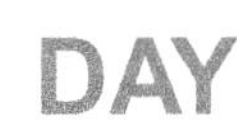 SLEEP   WEIGHT

WORKOUT ACTIVITIES / EXERCISES	SET / REPS / DISTANCE	CALORIES BURNED	TIME SPENT

NOTES/TODAY'S ACHIEVEMENT	WHAT WILL DO BETTER TOMORROW

M T W T F S S   MOOD 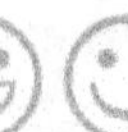   **DAY** 16

DATE ....

TODAY'S COMMITMENTS

____

____

TODAY MEALS	BREAKFAST	LUNCH	DINNER	SNACKS
	Calories:	Calories:	Calories:	Calories:

FATS	CARBS	PROTEINS	OTHERS

WATER ☐ ☐ ☐ ☐ ☐ ☐ ☐ ☐   SLEEP   WEIGHT

WORKOUT ACTIVITIES / EXERCISES	SET / REPS / DISTANCE	CALORIES BURNED	TIME SPENT

NOTES/TODAY'S ACHIEVEMENT	WHAT WILL DO BETTER TOMORROW

M T W T F S S   MOOD 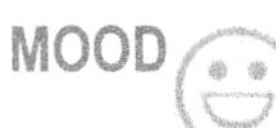   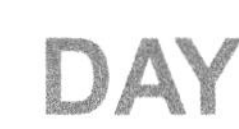 **DAY** | 17

DATE ....

TODAY'S COMMITMENTS

TODAY MEALS	BREAKFAST	LUNCH	DINNER	SNACKS
	Calories:	Calories:	Calories:	Calories:

FATS	CARBS	PROTEINS	OTHERS

WATER 🥛🥛🥛🥛🥛🥛🥛🥛 | SLEEP | WEIGHT

WORKOUT ACTIVITIES / EXERCISES	SET / REPS / DISTANCE	CALORIES BURNED	TIME SPENT

NOTES/TODAY'S ACHIEVEMENT	WHAT WILL DO BETTER TOMORROW

M T W T F S S   MOOD  

DAY 18

DATE ....

TODAY'S COMMITMENTS

	BREAKFAST	LUNCH	DINNER	SNACKS
TODAY MEALS				
	Calories:	Calories:	Calories:	Calories:

FATS	CARBS	PROTEINS	OTHERS

WATER 🥛🥛🥛🥛🥛🥛🥛🥛   SLEEP   WEIGHT

WORKOUT ACTIVITIES / EXERCISES	SET / REPS / DISTANCE	CALORIES BURNED	TIME SPENT

NOTES/TODAY'S ACHIEVEMENT	WHAT WILL DO BETTER TOMORROW

M T W T F S S   MOOD    **DAY** | 19

DATE ....

TODAY'S COMMITMENTS

____

____

	BREAKFAST	LUNCH	DINNER	SNACKS
TODAY MEALS				
	Calories:	Calories:	Calories:	Calories:

FATS	CARBS	PROTEINS	OTHERS

WATER ⬜ ⬜ ⬜ ⬜ ⬜ ⬜ ⬜ ⬜   SLEEP   WEIGHT

WORKOUT ACTIVITIES / EXERCISES	SET / REPS / DISTANCE	CALORIES BURNED	TIME SPENT

NOTES/TODAY'S ACHIEVEMENT	WHAT WILL DO BETTER TOMORROW

M T W T F S S   MOOD      **DAY | 20**

DATE ....

TODAY'S COMMITMENTS

	BREAKFAST	LUNCH	DINNER	SNACKS
TODAY MEALS				
	Calories:	Calories:	Calories:	Calories:

FATS	CARBS	PROTEINS	OTHERS

WATER 🥤🥤🥤🥤🥤🥤🥤🥤   ⏰ SLEEP   WEIGHT

WORKOUT ACTIVITIES / EXERCISES	SET / REPS / DISTANCE	CALORIES BURNED	TIME SPENT

NOTES/TODAY'S ACHIEVEMENT	WHAT WILL DO BETTER TOMORROW

M T W T F S S   MOOD   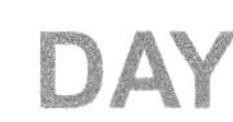 **DAY** | 21

DATE ....

TODAY'S COMMITMENTS

<table>
<tr><td rowspan="7">TODAY MEALS</td><td>BREAKFAST</td><td>LUNCH</td><td>DINNER</td><td>SNACKS</td></tr>
<tr><td></td><td></td><td></td><td></td></tr>
<tr><td></td><td></td><td></td><td></td></tr>
<tr><td></td><td></td><td></td><td></td></tr>
<tr><td></td><td></td><td></td><td></td></tr>
<tr><td></td><td></td><td></td><td></td></tr>
<tr><td>Calories:</td><td>Calories:</td><td>Calories:</td><td>Calories:</td></tr>
</table>

FATS	CARBS	PROTEINS	OTHERS

WATER ☐ ☐ ☐ ☐ ☐ ☐ ☐ ☐   SLEEP   WEIGHT

WORKOUT ACTIVITIES / EXERCISES	SET / REPS / DISTANCE	CALORIES BURNED	TIME SPENT

NOTES/TODAY'S ACHIEVEMENT	WHAT WILL DO BETTER TOMORROW

M T W T F S S   MOOD     **DAY** 22

DATE ....

TODAY'S COMMITMENTS

TODAY MEALS	BREAKFAST	LUNCH	DINNER	SNACKS
	Calories:	Calories:	Calories:	Calories:

FATS	CARBS	PROTEINS	OTHERS

WATER 🥛🥛🥛🥛🥛🥛🥛🥛   SLEEP   WEIGHT

WORKOUT ACTIVITIES / EXERCISES	SET / REPS / DISTANCE	CALORIES BURNED	TIME SPENT

NOTES/TODAY'S ACHIEVEMENT	WHAT WILL DO BETTER TOMORROW

M T W T F S S   MOOD   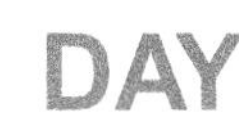   **DAY** 23

DATE ....

TODAY'S COMMITMENTS

TODAY MEALS	BREAKFAST	LUNCH	DINNER	SNACKS
	Calories:	Calories:	Calories:	Calories:

FATS	CARBS	PROTEINS	OTHERS

WATER

SLEEP

WEIGHT

WORKOUT ACTIVITIES / EXERCISES	SET / REPS / DISTANCE	CALORIES BURNED	TIME SPENT

NOTES/TODAY'S ACHIEVEMENT	WHAT WILL DO BETTER TOMORROW

M T W T F S S   MOOD    **DAY** | 24

DATE ....

TODAY'S COMMITMENTS

____

____

TODAY MEALS	BREAKFAST	LUNCH	DINNER	SNACKS
	Calories:	Calories:	Calories:	Calories:

FATS	CARBS	PROTEINS	OTHERS

WATER ⎕ ⎕ ⎕ ⎕ ⎕ ⎕ ⎕ ⎕   SLEEP   WEIGHT

WORKOUT ACTIVITIES / EXERCISES	SET / REPS / DISTANCE	CALORIES BURNED	TIME SPENT

NOTES/TODAY'S ACHIEVEMENT	WHAT WILL DO BETTER TOMORROW

M T W T F S S   MOOD 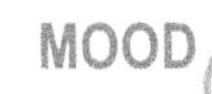 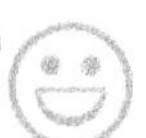   **DAY** | 25

DATE ....

TODAY'S COMMITMENTS

TODAY MEALS	BREAKFAST	LUNCH	DINNER	SNACKS
	Calories:	Calories:	Calories:	Calories:

FATS	CARBS	PROTEINS	OTHERS

WATER 🥛🥛🥛🥛🥛🥛🥛🥛   SLEEP   WEIGHT

WORKOUT ACTIVITIES / EXERCISES	SET / REPS / DISTANCE	CALORIES BURNED	TIME SPENT

NOTES/TODAY'S ACHIEVEMENT	WHAT WILL DO BETTER TOMORROW

M T W T F S S   MOOD     **DAY** 26

DATE ....

TODAY'S COMMITMENTS

	BREAKFAST	LUNCH	DINNER	SNACKS
TODAY MEALS				
	Calories:	Calories:	Calories:	Calories:

FATS	CARBS	PROTEINS	OTHERS

WATER ☐☐☐☐☐☐☐☐   SLEEP   WEIGHT

WORKOUT ACTIVITIES / EXERCISES	SET / REPS / DISTANCE	CALORIES BURNED	TIME SPENT

NOTES/TODAY'S ACHIEVEMENT	WHAT WILL DO BETTER TOMORROW

M T W T F S S   MOOD 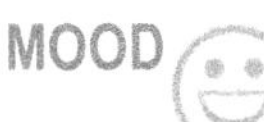   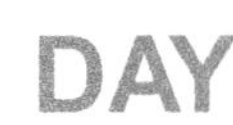   **DAY** | 27

DATE ....

TODAY'S COMMITMENTS

	BREAKFAST	LUNCH	DINNER	SNACKS
TODAY MEALS				
	Calories:	Calories:	Calories:	Calories:

FATS	CARBS	PROTEINS	OTHERS

WATER ☐ ☐ ☐ ☐ ☐ ☐ ☐ ☐   🕐 SLEEP   👣 WEIGHT

WORKOUT ACTIVITIES / EXERCISES	SET / REPS / DISTANCE	CALORIES BURNED	TIME SPENT

NOTES/TODAY'S ACHIEVEMENT	WHAT WILL DO BETTER TOMORROW

M T W T F S S   MOOD   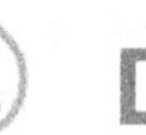   **DAY 28**

DATE ....

TODAY'S COMMITMENTS

TODAY MEALS	BREAKFAST	LUNCH	DINNER	SNACKS
	Calories:	Calories:	Calories:	Calories:

FATS	CARBS	PROTEINS	OTHERS

WATER □□□□□□□□   SLEEP   WEIGHT

WORKOUT ACTIVITIES / EXERCISES	SET / REPS / DISTANCE	CALORIES BURNED	TIME SPENT

NOTES/TODAY'S ACHIEVEMENT	WHAT WILL DO BETTER TOMORROW

M T W T F S S MOOD 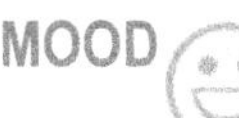   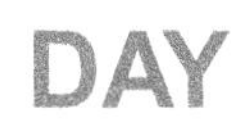 **DAY** | 29

DATE ....

TODAY'S COMMITMENTS

TODAY MEALS	BREAKFAST	LUNCH	DINNER	SNACKS
	Calories:	Calories:	Calories:	Calories:

FATS	CARBS	PROTEINS	OTHERS

WATER 🥤🥤🥤🥤🥤🥤🥤🥤 ⏰ SLEEP 👣 WEIGHT

WORKOUT ACTIVITIES / EXERCISES	SET / REPS / DISTANCE	CALORIES BURNED	TIME SPENT

NOTES/TODAY'S ACHIEVEMENT	WHAT WILL DO BETTER TOMORROW

TODAY'S COMMITMENTS

	BREAKFAST	LUNCH	DINNER	SNACKS
TODAY MEALS				
	Calories:	Calories:	Calories:	Calories:

FATS	CARBS	PROTEINS	OTHERS

WATER ☐ ☐ ☐ ☐ ☐ ☐ ☐ ☐   SLEEP   WEIGHT

WORKOUT ACTIVITIES / EXERCISES	SET / REPS / DISTANCE	CALORIES BURNED	TIME SPENT

NOTES/TODAY'S ACHIEVEMENT	WHAT WILL DO BETTER TOMORROW

M T W T F S S   MOOD 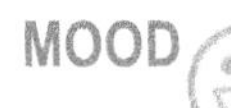  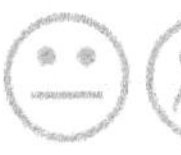 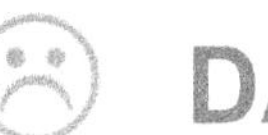   **DAY** | 31

DATE ....

TODAY'S COMMITMENTS

TODAY MEALS	BREAKFAST	LUNCH	DINNER	SNACKS
	Calories:	Calories:	Calories:	Calories:

FATS	CARBS	PROTEINS	OTHERS

WATER ☐ ☐ ☐ ☐ ☐ ☐ ☐ ☐   SLEEP   WEIGHT

WORKOUT ACTIVITIES / EXERCISES	SET / REPS / DISTANCE	CALORIES BURNED	TIME SPENT

NOTES/TODAY'S ACHIEVEMENT	WHAT WILL DO BETTER TOMORROW

M T W T F S S   MOOD      **DAY** | 32

DATE ....

TODAY'S COMMITMENTS

____

____

TODAY MEALS	BREAKFAST	LUNCH	DINNER	SNACKS
	Calories:	Calories:	Calories:	Calories:

FATS	CARBS	PROTEINS	OTHERS

WATER ⬜⬜⬜⬜⬜⬜⬜⬜   ⏰ SLEEP   WEIGHT

WORKOUT ACTIVITIES / EXERCISES	SET / REPS / DISTANCE	CALORIES BURNED	TIME SPENT

NOTES/TODAY'S ACHIEVEMENT	WHAT WILL DO BETTER TOMORROW

M T W T F S S   MOOD  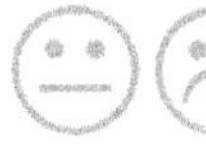   **DAY** 33

DATE ....

TODAY'S COMMITMENTS

<table>
<tr><th rowspan="2">TODAY MEALS</th><th>BREAKFAST</th><th>LUNCH</th><th>DINNER</th><th>SNACKS</th></tr>
<tr><td>Calories:</td><td>Calories:</td><td>Calories:</td><td>Calories:</td></tr>
</table>

FATS	CARBS	PROTEINS	OTHERS

WATER   SLEEP   WEIGHT

WORKOUT ACTIVITIES / EXERCISES	SET / REPS / DISTANCE	CALORIES BURNED	TIME SPENT

NOTES/TODAY'S ACHIEVEMENT	WHAT WILL DO BETTER TOMORROW

M T W T F S S   MOOD 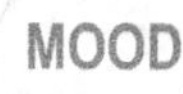     **DAY** | 34

DATE ....

TODAY'S COMMITMENTS

<table>
<tr><td rowspan="2">TODAY MEALS</td><td>BREAKFAST</td><td>LUNCH</td><td>DINNER</td><td>SNACKS</td></tr>
<tr><td>Calories:</td><td>Calories:</td><td>Calories:</td><td>Calories:</td></tr>
</table>

FATS	CARBS	PROTEINS	OTHERS

WATER 〔 〕〔 〕〔 〕〔 〕〔 〕〔 〕〔 〕〔 〕   SLEEP   WEIGHT

WORKOUT ACTIVITIES / EXERCISES	SET / REPS / DISTANCE	CALORIES BURNED	TIME SPENT

NOTES/TODAY'S ACHIEVEMENT	WHAT WILL DO BETTER TOMORROW

M T W T F S S   MOOD     **DAY** | 35

DATE ....

TODAY'S COMMITMENTS

<table>
<tr><td rowspan="7">TODAY MEALS</td><td>BREAKFAST</td><td>LUNCH</td><td>DINNER</td><td>SNACKS</td></tr>
<tr><td></td><td></td><td></td><td></td></tr>
<tr><td></td><td></td><td></td><td></td></tr>
<tr><td></td><td></td><td></td><td></td></tr>
<tr><td></td><td></td><td></td><td></td></tr>
<tr><td></td><td></td><td></td><td></td></tr>
<tr><td>Calories:</td><td>Calories:</td><td>Calories:</td><td>Calories:</td></tr>
</table>

FATS	CARBS	PROTEINS	OTHERS

WATER 🥤🥤🥤🥤🥤🥤🥤🥤   ⏰ SLEEP   👣 WEIGHT

WORKOUT ACTIVITIES / EXERCISES	SET / REPS / DISTANCE	CALORIES BURNED	TIME SPENT

NOTES/TODAY'S ACHIEVEMENT	WHAT WILL DO BETTER TOMORROW

M T W T F S S   MOOD      **DAY** 36

DATE ....

TODAY'S COMMITMENTS

TODAY MEALS	BREAKFAST	LUNCH	DINNER	SNACKS
	Calories:	Calories:	Calories:	Calories:

FATS	CARBS	PROTEINS	OTHERS

WATER   ⬚ ⬚ ⬚ ⬚ ⬚ ⬚ ⬚ ⬚   SLEEP   WEIGHT

WORKOUT ACTIVITIES / EXERCISES	SET / REPS / DISTANCE	CALORIES BURNED	TIME SPENT

NOTES/TODAY'S ACHIEVEMENT	WHAT WILL DO BETTER TOMORROW

M T W T F S S   MOOD 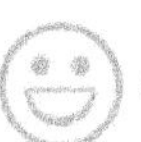     **DAY** | 37

DATE ....

TODAY'S COMMITMENTS

TODAY MEALS	BREAKFAST	LUNCH	DINNER	SNACKS
	Calories:	Calories:	Calories:	Calories:

FATS	CARBS	PROTEINS	OTHERS

WATER ☐ ☐ ☐ ☐ ☐ ☐ ☐ ☐   SLEEP   WEIGHT

WORKOUT ACTIVITIES / EXERCISES	SET / REPS / DISTANCE	CALORIES BURNED	TIME SPENT

NOTES/TODAY'S ACHIEVEMENT	WHAT WILL DO BETTER TOMORROW

M T W T F S S   MOOD      DAY 38

DATE ....

TODAY'S COMMITMENTS

<table>
<tr><td rowspan="2">TODAY MEALS</td><td>BREAKFAST</td><td>LUNCH</td><td>DINNER</td><td>SNACKS</td></tr>
<tr><td>Calories:</td><td>Calories:</td><td>Calories:</td><td>Calories:</td></tr>
</table>

FATS	CARBS	PROTEINS	OTHERS

WATER 〇 〇 〇 〇 〇 〇 〇 〇   SLEEP   WEIGHT

WORKOUT ACTIVITIES / EXERCISES	SET / REPS / DISTANCE	CALORIES BURNED	TIME SPENT

NOTES/TODAY'S ACHIEVEMENT	WHAT WILL DO BETTER TOMORROW

M T W T F S S   MOOD     **DAY** | 39

DATE ....

TODAY'S COMMITMENTS

<table>
<tr><td rowspan="2">TODAY MEALS</td><td>BREAKFAST</td><td>LUNCH</td><td>DINNER</td><td>SNACKS</td></tr>
<tr><td>Calories:</td><td>Calories:</td><td>Calories:</td><td>Calories:</td></tr>
</table>

FATS	CARBS	PROTEINS	OTHERS

WATER SLEEP WEIGHT

WORKOUT ACTIVITIES / EXERCISES	SET / REPS / DISTANCE	CALORIES BURNED	TIME SPENT

NOTES/TODAY'S ACHIEVEMENT	WHAT WILL DO BETTER TOMORROW

M T W T F S S   MOOD   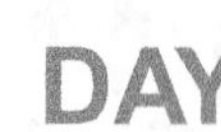   # DAY | 40

DATE ....

TODAY'S COMMITMENTS

<table>
<tr><th rowspan="2">TODAY MEALS</th><th>BREAKFAST</th><th>LUNCH</th><th>DINNER</th><th>SNACKS</th></tr>
<tr><td>Calories:</td><td>Calories:</td><td>Calories:</td><td>Calories:</td></tr>
</table>

FATS	CARBS	PROTEINS	OTHERS

WATER

SLEEP

WEIGHT

WORKOUT ACTIVITIES / EXERCISES	SET / REPS / DISTANCE	CALORIES BURNED	TIME SPENT

NOTES/TODAY'S ACHIEVEMENT	WHAT WILL DO BETTER TOMORROW

M T W T F S S   MOOD   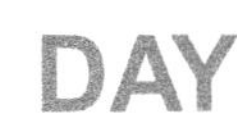   **DAY** | 41

DATE ....

TODAY'S COMMITMENTS

	BREAKFAST	LUNCH	DINNER	SNACKS
TODAY MEALS				
	Calories:	Calories:	Calories:	Calories:

FATS	CARBS	PROTEINS	OTHERS

WATER ⬜⬜⬜⬜⬜⬜⬜⬜   SLEEP   WEIGHT

WORKOUT ACTIVITIES / EXERCISES	SET / REPS / DISTANCE	CALORIES BURNED	TIME SPENT

NOTES/TODAY'S ACHIEVEMENT	WHAT WILL DO BETTER TOMORROW

M T W T F S S MOOD    **DAY** 42

DATE ....

TODAY'S COMMITMENTS

TODAY MEALS	BREAKFAST	LUNCH	DINNER	SNACKS
	Calories:	Calories:	Calories:	Calories:

FATS	CARBS	PROTEINS	OTHERS

WATER 🥛🥛🥛🥛🥛🥛🥛🥛   ⏰ SLEEP   👣 WEIGHT

WORKOUT ACTIVITIES / EXERCISES	SET / REPS / DISTANCE	CALORIES BURNED	TIME SPENT

NOTES/TODAY'S ACHIEVEMENT	WHAT WILL DO BETTER TOMORROW

M T W T F S S   MOOD  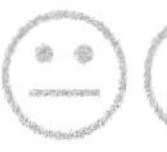 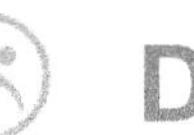 **DAY** 43

DATE ....

TODAY'S COMMITMENTS

____

____

TODAY MEALS	BREAKFAST	LUNCH	DINNER	SNACKS
	Calories:	Calories:	Calories:	Calories:

FATS	CARBS	PROTEINS	OTHERS

WATER ⬜⬜⬜⬜⬜⬜⬜⬜   SLEEP   WEIGHT

WORKOUT ACTIVITIES / EXERCISES	SET / REPS / DISTANCE	CALORIES BURNED	TIME SPENT

NOTES/TODAY'S ACHIEVEMENT	WHAT WILL DO BETTER TOMORROW

M T W T F S S   MOOD     **DAY** 44

DATE ....

TODAY'S COMMITMENTS

____

____

____

TODAY MEALS	BREAKFAST	LUNCH	DINNER	SNACKS
	Calories:	Calories:	Calories:	Calories:

FATS	CARBS	PROTEINS	OTHERS

WATER ⬜⬜⬜⬜⬜⬜⬜⬜   SLEEP   WEIGHT

WORKOUT ACTIVITIES / EXERCISES	SET / REPS / DISTANCE	CALORIES BURNED	TIME SPENT

NOTES/TODAY'S ACHIEVEMENT	WHAT WILL DO BETTER TOMORROW

M T W T F S S   MOOD 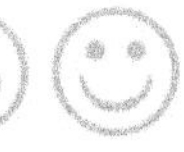  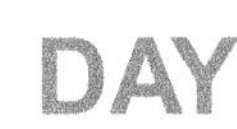   **DAY** | 45

DATE ....

TODAY'S COMMITMENTS

	BREAKFAST	LUNCH	DINNER	SNACKS
TODAY MEALS				
	Calories:	Calories:	Calories:	Calories:

FATS	CARBS	PROTEINS	OTHERS

WATER ▢ ▢ ▢ ▢ ▢ ▢ ▢ ▢   SLEEP   WEIGHT

WORKOUT ACTIVITIES / EXERCISES	SET / REPS / DISTANCE	CALORIES BURNED	TIME SPENT

NOTES/TODAY'S ACHIEVEMENT	WHAT WILL DO BETTER TOMORROW

M T W T F S S   MOOD   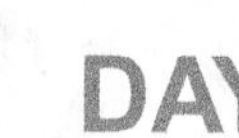 **DAY** 46

DATE ....

TODAY'S COMMITMENTS

____

____

TODAY MEALS	BREAKFAST	LUNCH	DINNER	SNACKS
	Calories:	Calories:	Calories:	Calories:

FATS	CARBS	PROTEINS	OTHERS

WATER [ ] [ ] [ ] [ ] [ ] [ ] [ ] [ ]   SLEEP   WEIGHT

WORKOUT ACTIVITIES / EXERCISES	SET / REPS / DISTANCE	CALORIES BURNED	TIME SPENT

NOTES/TODAY'S ACHIEVEMENT	WHAT WILL DO BETTER TOMORROW

M T W T F S S   MOOD 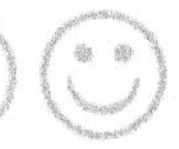    **DAY** | 47

DATE ....

TODAY'S COMMITMENTS

TODAY MEALS	BREAKFAST	LUNCH	DINNER	SNACKS
	Calories:	Calories:	Calories:	Calories:

FATS	CARBS	PROTEINS	OTHERS

WATER

SLEEP

WEIGHT

WORKOUT ACTIVITIES / EXERCISES	SET / REPS / DISTANCE	CALORIES BURNED	TIME SPENT

NOTES/TODAY'S ACHIEVEMENT	WHAT WILL DO BETTER TOMORROW

M T W T F S S   MOOD     # DAY | 48

DATE ....

TODAY'S COMMITMENTS

	BREAKFAST	LUNCH	DINNER	SNACKS
TODAY MEALS				
	Calories:	Calories:	Calories:	Calories:

FATS	CARBS	PROTEINS	OTHERS

WATER ☐ ☐ ☐ ☐ ☐ ☐ ☐ ☐   SLEEP   WEIGHT

WORKOUT ACTIVITIES / EXERCISES	SET / REPS / DISTANCE	CALORIES BURNED	TIME SPENT

NOTES/TODAY'S ACHIEVEMENT	WHAT WILL DO BETTER TOMORROW

M T W T F S S   MOOD      **DAY** 49

DATE ....

TODAY'S COMMITMENTS

TODAY MEALS	BREAKFAST	LUNCH	DINNER	SNACKS
	Calories:	Calories:	Calories:	Calories:

FATS	CARBS	PROTEINS	OTHERS

WATER ☐ ☐ ☐ ☐ ☐ ☐ ☐ ☐   ⏰ SLEEP   WEIGHT

WORKOUT ACTIVITIES / EXERCISES	SET / REPS / DISTANCE	CALORIES BURNED	TIME SPENT

NOTES/TODAY'S ACHIEVEMENT	WHAT WILL DO BETTER TOMORROW

M T W T F S S   MOOD   **DAY** 50

DATE ....

TODAY'S COMMITMENTS

TODAY MEALS	BREAKFAST	LUNCH	DINNER	SNACKS
	Calories:	Calories:	Calories:	Calories:

FATS	CARBS	PROTEINS	OTHERS

WATER ☐ ☐ ☐ ☐ ☐ ☐ ☐ ☐   SLEEP   WEIGHT

WORKOUT ACTIVITIES / EXERCISES	SET / REPS / DISTANCE	CALORIES BURNED	TIME SPENT

NOTES/TODAY'S ACHIEVEMENT	WHAT WILL DO BETTER TOMORROW

M T W T F S S   MOOD   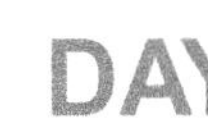   **DAY** 51

DATE ....

TODAY'S COMMITMENTS

TODAY MEALS	BREAKFAST	LUNCH	DINNER	SNACKS
	Calories:	Calories:	Calories:	Calories:

FATS	CARBS	PROTEINS	OTHERS

WATER · SLEEP · WEIGHT

WORKOUT ACTIVITIES / EXERCISES	SET / REPS / DISTANCE	CALORIES BURNED	TIME SPENT

NOTES/TODAY'S ACHIEVEMENT	WHAT WILL DO BETTER TOMORROW

M T W T F S S   MOOD     **DAY** 52

DATE ....

TODAY'S COMMITMENTS

TODAY MEALS	BREAKFAST	LUNCH	DINNER	SNACKS
	Calories:	Calories:	Calories:	Calories:

FATS	CARBS	PROTEINS	OTHERS

WATER SLEEP WEIGHT

WORKOUT ACTIVITIES / EXERCISES	SET / REPS / DISTANCE	CALORIES BURNED	TIME SPENT

NOTES/TODAY'S ACHIEVEMENT	WHAT WILL DO BETTER TOMORROW

M T W T F S S   MOOD 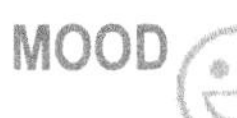  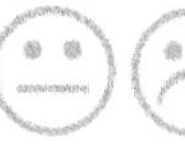 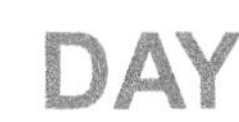   **DAY** | 53

DATE ....

TODAY'S COMMITMENTS

	BREAKFAST	LUNCH	DINNER	SNACKS
TODAY MEALS				
	Calories:	Calories:	Calories:	Calories:

FATS	CARBS	PROTEINS	OTHERS

WATER	SLEEP	WEIGHT

WORKOUT ACTIVITIES / EXERCISES	SET / REPS / DISTANCE	CALORIES BURNED	TIME SPENT

NOTES/TODAY'S ACHIEVEMENT	WHAT WILL DO BETTER TOMORROW

DAY 54

DATE ....

TODAY'S COMMITMENTS

____

____

TODAY MEALS	BREAKFAST	LUNCH	DINNER	SNACKS
	Calories:	Calories:	Calories:	Calories:

FATS	CARBS	PROTEINS	OTHERS

WATER 🥤🥤🥤🥤🥤🥤🥤🥤 ⏰ SLEEP ⚖ WEIGHT

WORKOUT ACTIVITIES / EXERCISES	SET / REPS / DISTANCE	CALORIES BURNED	TIME SPENT

NOTES/TODAY'S ACHIEVEMENT	WHAT WILL DO BETTER TOMORROW

M T W T F S S MOOD 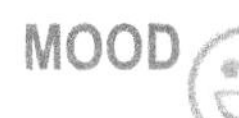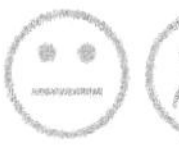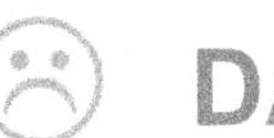 **DAY** 55

DATE ....

TODAY'S COMMITMENTS

	BREAKFAST	LUNCH	DINNER	SNACKS
TODAY MEALS				
	Calories:	Calories:	Calories:	Calories:

FATS	CARBS	PROTEINS	OTHERS

WATER ☐ ☐ ☐ ☐ ☐ ☐ ☐ ☐   SLEEP   WEIGHT

WORKOUT ACTIVITIES / EXERCISES	SET / REPS / DISTANCE	CALORIES BURNED	TIME SPENT

NOTES/TODAY'S ACHIEVEMENT	WHAT WILL DO BETTER TOMORROW

M T W T F S S   MOOD 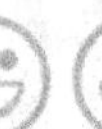     **DAY** | 56

DATE ....

TODAY'S COMMITMENTS

____

____

____

TODAY MEALS	BREAKFAST	LUNCH	DINNER	SNACKS
	Calories:	Calories:	Calories:	Calories:

FATS	CARBS	PROTEINS	OTHERS

WATER ⬜⬜⬜⬜⬜⬜⬜⬜   SLEEP   WEIGHT

WORKOUT ACTIVITIES / EXERCISES	SET / REPS / DISTANCE	CALORIES BURNED	TIME SPENT

NOTES/TODAY'S ACHIEVEMENT	WHAT WILL DO BETTER TOMORROW

M T W T F S S   MOOD 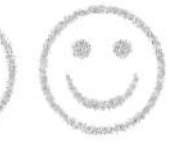  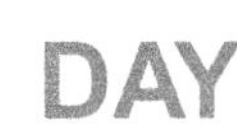   **DAY** | 57

DATE ....

TODAY'S COMMITMENTS

<table>
<tr><th rowspan="2">TODAY MEALS</th><th>BREAKFAST</th><th>LUNCH</th><th>DINNER</th><th>SNACKS</th></tr>
<tr><td>Calories:</td><td>Calories:</td><td>Calories:</td><td>Calories:</td></tr>
</table>

FATS	CARBS	PROTEINS	OTHERS

WATER   SLEEP   WEIGHT

WORKOUT ACTIVITIES / EXERCISES	SET / REPS / DISTANCE	CALORIES BURNED	TIME SPENT

NOTES/TODAY'S ACHIEVEMENT	WHAT WILL DO BETTER TOMORROW

M T W T F S S MOOD 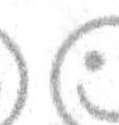   **DAY** 58

DATE ....

TODAY'S COMMITMENTS

____

____

TODAY MEALS	BREAKFAST	LUNCH	DINNER	SNACKS
	Calories:	Calories:	Calories:	Calories:

FATS	CARBS	PROTEINS	OTHERS

WATER 🥤🥤🥤🥤🥤🥤🥤🥤   ⏰ SLEEP   👣 WEIGHT

WORKOUT ACTIVITIES / EXERCISES	SET / REPS / DISTANCE	CALORIES BURNED	TIME SPENT

NOTES/TODAY'S ACHIEVEMENT	WHAT WILL DO BETTER TOMORROW

TODAY'S COMMITMENTS

TODAY MEALS	BREAKFAST	LUNCH	DINNER	SNACKS
	Calories:	Calories:	Calories:	Calories:

FATS	CARBS	PROTEINS	OTHERS

WATER ⎰⎰⎰⎰⎰⎰⎰⎰   🕐 SLEEP   👣 WEIGHT

WORKOUT ACTIVITIES / EXERCISES	SET / REPS / DISTANCE	CALORIES BURNED	TIME SPENT

NOTES/TODAY'S ACHIEVEMENT	WHAT WILL DO BETTER TOMORROW

TODAY'S COMMITMENTS

TODAY MEALS	BREAKFAST	LUNCH	DINNER	SNACKS
	Calories:	Calories:	Calories:	Calories:

FATS	CARBS	PROTEINS	OTHERS

WATER ⊔ ⊔ ⊔ ⊔ ⊔ ⊔ ⊔ ⊔   SLEEP   WEIGHT

WORKOUT ACTIVITIES / EXERCISES	SET / REPS / DISTANCE	CALORIES BURNED	TIME SPENT

NOTES/TODAY'S ACHIEVEMENT	WHAT WILL DO BETTER TOMORROW

M T W T F S S   MOOD    **DAY** 61

DATE ....

TODAY'S COMMITMENTS

<table>
<tr><th rowspan="2">TODAY MEALS</th><th>BREAKFAST</th><th>LUNCH</th><th>DINNER</th><th>SNACKS</th></tr>
<tr><td>Calories:</td><td>Calories:</td><td>Calories:</td><td>Calories:</td></tr>
</table>

FATS	CARBS	PROTEINS	OTHERS

WATER ⬜⬜⬜⬜⬜⬜⬜⬜   SLEEP   WEIGHT

WORKOUT ACTIVITIES / EXERCISES	SET / REPS / DISTANCE	CALORIES BURNED	TIME SPENT

NOTES/TODAY'S ACHIEVEMENT	WHAT WILL DO BETTER TOMORROW

M T W T F S S   MOOD    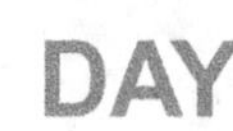   **DAY** 62

DATE ....

TODAY'S COMMITMENTS

____

____

____

TODAY MEALS	BREAKFAST	LUNCH	DINNER	SNACKS
	Calories:	Calories:	Calories:	Calories:

FATS	CARBS	PROTEINS	OTHERS

WATER 🥛🥛🥛🥛🥛🥛🥛🥛   SLEEP   WEIGHT

WORKOUT ACTIVITIES / EXERCISES	SET / REPS / DISTANCE	CALORIES BURNED	TIME SPENT

NOTES/TODAY'S ACHIEVEMENT	WHAT WILL DO BETTER TOMORROW

TODAY'S COMMITMENTS

TODAY MEALS	BREAKFAST	LUNCH	DINNER	SNACKS
	Calories:	Calories:	Calories:	Calories:

FATS	CARBS	PROTEINS	OTHERS

WATER ☐ ☐ ☐ ☐ ☐ ☐ ☐ ☐   SLEEP   WEIGHT

WORKOUT ACTIVITIES / EXERCISES	SET / REPS / DISTANCE	CALORIES BURNED	TIME SPENT

NOTES/TODAY'S ACHIEVEMENT	WHAT WILL DO BETTER TOMORROW

M T W T F S S   MOOD      **DAY** | 64

DATE ....

TODAY'S COMMITMENTS

TODAY MEALS	BREAKFAST	LUNCH	DINNER	SNACKS
	Calories:	Calories:	Calories:	Calories:

FATS	CARBS	PROTEINS	OTHERS

WATER ☐ ☐ ☐ ☐ ☐ ☐ ☐ ☐   SLEEP   WEIGHT

WORKOUT ACTIVITIES / EXERCISES	SET / REPS / DISTANCE	CALORIES BURNED	TIME SPENT

NOTES/TODAY'S ACHIEVEMENT	WHAT WILL DO BETTER TOMORROW

M T W T F S S   MOOD 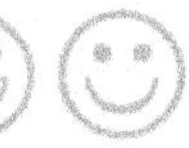 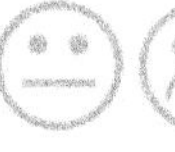   **DAY** | 65

DATE ....

TODAY'S COMMITMENTS

TODAY MEALS	BREAKFAST	LUNCH	DINNER	SNACKS
	Calories:	Calories:	Calories:	Calories:

FATS	CARBS	PROTEINS	OTHERS

WATER ⬜⬜⬜⬜⬜⬜⬜⬜   ⏰ SLEEP   WEIGHT

WORKOUT ACTIVITIES / EXERCISES	SET / REPS / DISTANCE	CALORIES BURNED	TIME SPENT

NOTES/TODAY'S ACHIEVEMENT	WHAT WILL DO BETTER TOMORROW

M T W T F S S   MOOD 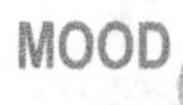   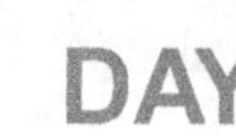   **DAY** | 66

DATE ....

TODAY'S COMMITMENTS

____

____

<table>
<tr><td rowspan="2">TODAY MEALS</td><td>BREAKFAST</td><td>LUNCH</td><td>DINNER</td><td>SNACKS</td></tr>
<tr><td>Calories:</td><td>Calories:</td><td>Calories:</td><td>Calories:</td></tr>
</table>

FATS	CARBS	PROTEINS	OTHERS

WATER ⬜⬜⬜⬜⬜⬜⬜⬜   🕐 SLEEP   WEIGHT

WORKOUT ACTIVITIES / EXERCISES	SET / REPS / DISTANCE	CALORIES BURNED	TIME SPENT

NOTES/TODAY'S ACHIEVEMENT	WHAT WILL DO BETTER TOMORROW

M T W T F S S   MOOD 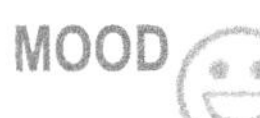     **DAY** | 67

DATE ....

TODAY'S COMMITMENTS

<table>
<tr><td rowspan="2">TODAY MEALS</td><td>BREAKFAST</td><td>LUNCH</td><td>DINNER</td><td>SNACKS</td></tr>
<tr><td>Calories:</td><td>Calories:</td><td>Calories:</td><td>Calories:</td></tr>
</table>

FATS	CARBS	PROTEINS	OTHERS

WATER ☐ ☐ ☐ ☐ ☐ ☐ ☐ ☐   SLEEP   WEIGHT

WORKOUT ACTIVITIES / EXERCISES	SET / REPS / DISTANCE	CALORIES BURNED	TIME SPENT

NOTES/TODAY'S ACHIEVEMENT	WHAT WILL DO BETTER TOMORROW

M T W T F S S   MOOD 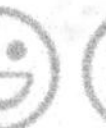     **DAY** 68

DATE ....

TODAY'S COMMITMENTS

____

____

____

TODAY MEALS	BREAKFAST	LUNCH	DINNER	SNACKS
	Calories:	Calories:	Calories:	Calories:

FATS	CARBS	PROTEINS	OTHERS

WATER ⬜⬜⬜⬜⬜⬜⬜⬜   🕐 SLEEP   WEIGHT

WORKOUT ACTIVITIES / EXERCISES	SET / REPS / DISTANCE	CALORIES BURNED	TIME SPENT

NOTES/TODAY'S ACHIEVEMENT	WHAT WILL DO BETTER TOMORROW

M T W T F S S MOOD    **DAY** 69

DATE ....

TODAY'S COMMITMENTS

<table>
<tr><td rowspan="2">TODAY MEALS</td><td>BREAKFAST</td><td>LUNCH</td><td>DINNER</td><td>SNACKS</td></tr>
<tr><td>Calories:</td><td>Calories:</td><td>Calories:</td><td>Calories:</td></tr>
</table>

FATS	CARBS	PROTEINS	OTHERS

WATER □ □ □ □ □ □ □ □   SLEEP   WEIGHT

WORKOUT ACTIVITIES / EXERCISES	SET / REPS / DISTANCE	CALORIES BURNED	TIME SPENT

NOTES/TODAY'S ACHIEVEMENT	WHAT WILL DO BETTER TOMORROW

MOOD 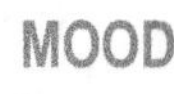  

DAY 70

DATE ....

TODAY'S COMMITMENTS

____

____

TODAY MEALS	BREAKFAST	LUNCH	DINNER	SNACKS
	Calories:	Calories:	Calories:	Calories:

FATS	CARBS	PROTEINS	OTHERS

WATER SLEEP WEIGHT

WORKOUT ACTIVITIES / EXERCISES	SET / REPS / DISTANCE	CALORIES BURNED	TIME SPENT

NOTES/TODAY'S ACHIEVEMENT	WHAT WILL DO BETTER TOMORROW

M T W T F S S   MOOD  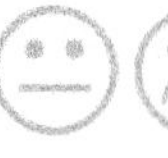   **DAY** | 71

DATE ....

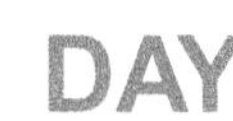

TODAY'S COMMITMENTS

TODAY MEALS	BREAKFAST	LUNCH	DINNER	SNACKS
	Calories:	Calories:	Calories:	Calories:

FATS	CARBS	PROTEINS	OTHERS

WATER ⎕ ⎕ ⎕ ⎕ ⎕ ⎕ ⎕ ⎕   ⏰ SLEEP   WEIGHT

WORKOUT ACTIVITIES / EXERCISES	SET / REPS / DISTANCE	CALORIES BURNED	TIME SPENT

NOTES/TODAY'S ACHIEVEMENT	WHAT WILL DO BETTER TOMORROW

M T W T F S S   MOOD   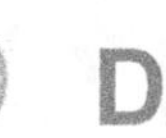   **DAY** | 72

DATE ....

TODAY'S COMMITMENTS

____

____

TODAY MEALS	BREAKFAST	LUNCH	DINNER	SNACKS
	Calories:	Calories:	Calories:	Calories:

FATS	CARBS	PROTEINS	OTHERS

WATER 🥤🥤🥤🥤🥤🥤🥤🥤 ⏰ SLEEP   👣 WEIGHT

WORKOUT ACTIVITIES / EXERCISES	SET / REPS / DISTANCE	CALORIES BURNED	TIME SPENT

NOTES/TODAY'S ACHIEVEMENT	WHAT WILL DO BETTER TOMORROW

M T W T F S S   MOOD 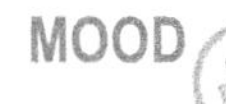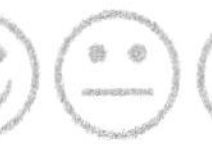   **DAY** 73

DATE ....

TODAY'S COMMITMENTS

<table>
<tr><td rowspan="2">TODAY MEALS</td><td>BREAKFAST</td><td>LUNCH</td><td>DINNER</td><td>SNACKS</td></tr>
<tr><td>Calories:</td><td>Calories:</td><td>Calories:</td><td>Calories:</td></tr>
</table>

FATS	CARBS	PROTEINS	OTHERS

WATER 🥤🥤🥤🥤🥤🥤🥤🥤   ⏰ SLEEP   👣 WEIGHT

WORKOUT ACTIVITIES / EXERCISES	SET / REPS / DISTANCE	CALORIES BURNED	TIME SPENT

NOTES/TODAY'S ACHIEVEMENT	WHAT WILL DO BETTER TOMORROW

M T W T F S S MOOD    **DAY 74**

DATE ....

TODAY'S COMMITMENTS

____

____

TODAY MEALS	BREAKFAST	LUNCH	DINNER	SNACKS
	Calories:	Calories:	Calories:	Calories:

FATS	CARBS	PROTEINS	OTHERS

WATER ☐ ☐ ☐ ☐ ☐ ☐ ☐ ☐   SLEEP   WEIGHT

WORKOUT ACTIVITIES / EXERCISES	SET / REPS / DISTANCE	CALORIES BURNED	TIME SPENT

NOTES/TODAY'S ACHIEVEMENT	WHAT WILL DO BETTER TOMORROW

MOOD 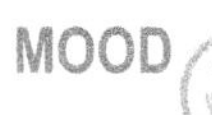 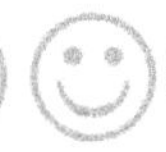  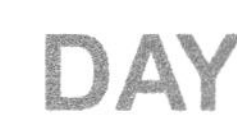

DATE ....

DAY | 75

TODAY'S COMMITMENTS

____

____

TODAY MEALS	BREAKFAST	LUNCH	DINNER	SNACKS
	Calories:	Calories:	Calories:	Calories:

FATS	CARBS	PROTEINS	OTHERS

WATER ⬜⬜⬜⬜⬜⬜⬜⬜ ⏰ SLEEP   WEIGHT

WORKOUT ACTIVITIES / EXERCISES	SET / REPS / DISTANCE	CALORIES BURNED	TIME SPENT

NOTES/TODAY'S ACHIEVEMENT	WHAT WILL DO BETTER TOMORROW

DATE ....

MOOD 

DAY | 76

TODAY'S COMMITMENTS

____

____

TODAY MEALS	BREAKFAST	LUNCH	DINNER	SNACKS
	Calories:	Calories:	Calories:	Calories:

FATS	CARBS	PROTEINS	OTHERS

WATER 🥛🥛🥛🥛🥛🥛🥛🥛 SLEEP WEIGHT

WORKOUT ACTIVITIES / EXERCISES	SET / REPS / DISTANCE	CALORIES BURNED	TIME SPENT

NOTES/TODAY'S ACHIEVEMENT	WHAT WILL DO BETTER TOMORROW

M T W T F S S   MOOD 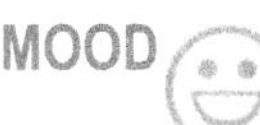   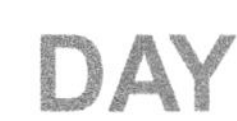   **DAY** 77

DATE ....

TODAY'S COMMITMENTS

TODAY MEALS	BREAKFAST	LUNCH	DINNER	SNACKS
Calories:	Calories:	Calories:	Calories:	

FATS	CARBS	PROTEINS	OTHERS

WATER 🥛🥛🥛🥛🥛🥛🥛🥛 ⏰ SLEEP WEIGHT

WORKOUT ACTIVITIES / EXERCISES	SET / REPS / DISTANCE	CALORIES BURNED	TIME SPENT

NOTES/TODAY'S ACHIEVEMENT	WHAT WILL DO BETTER TOMORROW

M T W T F S S   MOOD   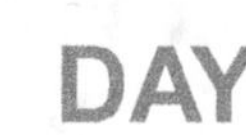   **DAY** 78

DATE ....

TODAY'S COMMITMENTS

____

____

TODAY MEALS	BREAKFAST	LUNCH	DINNER	SNACKS
	Calories:	Calories:	Calories:	Calories:

FATS	CARBS	PROTEINS	OTHERS

WATER 🥛🥛🥛🥛🥛🥛🥛🥛 ⏰ SLEEP WEIGHT

WORKOUT ACTIVITIES / EXERCISES	SET / REPS / DISTANCE	CALORIES BURNED	TIME SPENT

NOTES/TODAY'S ACHIEVEMENT	WHAT WILL DO BETTER TOMORROW

M T W T F S S   MOOD 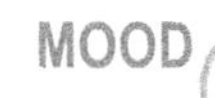   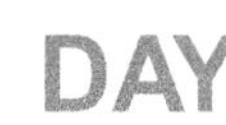   **DAY** | 79

DATE ....

TODAY'S COMMITMENTS

TODAY MEALS	BREAKFAST	LUNCH	DINNER	SNACKS
	Calories:	Calories:	Calories:	Calories:

FATS	CARBS	PROTEINS	OTHERS

WATER ☐ ☐ ☐ ☐ ☐ ☐ ☐ ☐   SLEEP   WEIGHT

WORKOUT ACTIVITIES / EXERCISES	SET / REPS / DISTANCE	CALORIES BURNED	TIME SPENT

NOTES/TODAY'S ACHIEVEMENT	WHAT WILL DO BETTER TOMORROW

M T W T F S S   MOOD   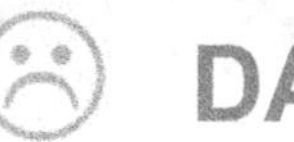 DAY | 80

DATE ....

TODAY'S COMMITMENTS

____

____

TODAY MEALS	BREAKFAST	LUNCH	DINNER	SNACKS
	Calories:	Calories:	Calories:	Calories:

FATS	CARBS	PROTEINS	OTHERS

WATER ⎕ ⎕ ⎕ ⎕ ⎕ ⎕ ⎕ ⎕   ⏰ SLEEP   WEIGHT

WORKOUT ACTIVITIES / EXERCISES	SET / REPS / DISTANCE	CALORIES BURNED	TIME SPENT

NOTES/TODAY'S ACHIEVEMENT	WHAT WILL DO BETTER TOMORROW

M T W T F S S   MOOD   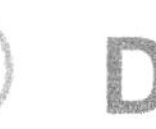 **DAY** | 81

DATE ....

TODAY'S COMMITMENTS

	BREAKFAST	LUNCH	DINNER	SNACKS
TODAY MEALS				
	Calories:	Calories:	Calories:	Calories:

FATS	CARBS	PROTEINS	OTHERS

WATER ☐ ☐ ☐ ☐ ☐ ☐ ☐ ☐   SLEEP   WEIGHT

WORKOUT ACTIVITIES / EXERCISES	SET / REPS / DISTANCE	CALORIES BURNED	TIME SPENT

NOTES/TODAY'S ACHIEVEMENT	WHAT WILL DO BETTER TOMORROW

M T W T F S S   MOOD      **DAY** | 82

DATE ....

TODAY'S COMMITMENTS

TODAY MEALS	BREAKFAST	LUNCH	DINNER	SNACKS
	Calories:	Calories:	Calories:	Calories:

FATS	CARBS	PROTEINS	OTHERS

WATER ▢ ▢ ▢ ▢ ▢ ▢ ▢ ▢   SLEEP   WEIGHT

WORKOUT ACTIVITIES / EXERCISES	SET / REPS / DISTANCE	CALORIES BURNED	TIME SPENT

NOTES/TODAY'S ACHIEVEMENT	WHAT WILL DO BETTER TOMORROW

M T W T F S S   MOOD  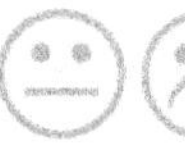   **DAY** | 83

DATE ....

TODAY'S COMMITMENTS

	BREAKFAST	LUNCH	DINNER	SNACKS
TODAY MEALS				
	Calories:	Calories:	Calories:	Calories:

FATS	CARBS	PROTEINS	OTHERS

WATER ⊔⊔⊔⊔⊔⊔⊔⊔	⏰ SLEEP	👣 WEIGHT

WORKOUT ACTIVITIES / EXERCISES	SET / REPS / DISTANCE	CALORIES BURNED	TIME SPENT

NOTES/TODAY'S ACHIEVEMENT	WHAT WILL DO BETTER TOMORROW

M T W T F S S   MOOD   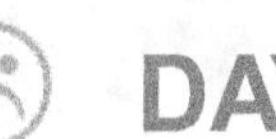   **DAY** | 84

DATE ....

TODAY'S COMMITMENTS

____

____

TODAY MEALS	BREAKFAST	LUNCH	DINNER	SNACKS
	Calories:	Calories:	Calories:	Calories:

FATS	CARBS	PROTEINS	OTHERS

WATER 🥛🥛🥛🥛🥛🥛🥛🥛   ⏰ SLEEP   👣 WEIGHT

WORKOUT ACTIVITIES / EXERCISES	SET / REPS / DISTANCE	CALORIES BURNED	TIME SPENT

NOTES/TODAY'S ACHIEVEMENT	WHAT WILL DO BETTER TOMORROW

M T W T F S S   MOOD 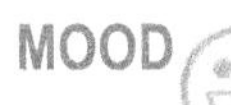 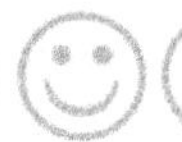 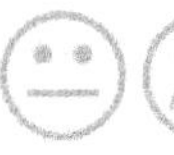    **DAY** | 85

DATE ....

TODAY'S COMMITMENTS

TODAY MEALS	BREAKFAST	LUNCH	DINNER	SNACKS
	Calories:	Calories:	Calories:	Calories:

FATS	CARBS	PROTEINS	OTHERS

WATER ⬜ ⬜ ⬜ ⬜ ⬜ ⬜ ⬜ ⬜   SLEEP   WEIGHT

WORKOUT ACTIVITIES / EXERCISES	SET / REPS / DISTANCE	CALORIES BURNED	TIME SPENT

NOTES/TODAY'S ACHIEVEMENT	WHAT WILL DO BETTER TOMORROW

M T W T F S S   MOOD 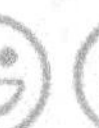     **DAY** 86

DATE ....

TODAY'S COMMITMENTS

TODAY MEALS	BREAKFAST	LUNCH	DINNER	SNACKS
	Calories:	Calories:	Calories:	Calories:

FATS	CARBS	PROTEINS	OTHERS

WATER ⬜⬜⬜⬜⬜⬜⬜⬜   SLEEP   WEIGHT

WORKOUT ACTIVITIES / EXERCISES	SET / REPS / DISTANCE	CALORIES BURNED	TIME SPENT

NOTES/TODAY'S ACHIEVEMENT	WHAT WILL DO BETTER TOMORROW

M T W T F S S   MOOD  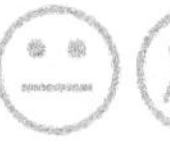   **DAY** 87

DATE ....

TODAY'S COMMITMENTS

____

____

<table>
<tr><td rowspan="2">TODAY MEALS</td><td>BREAKFAST</td><td>LUNCH</td><td>DINNER</td><td>SNACKS</td></tr>
<tr><td>Calories:</td><td>Calories:</td><td>Calories:</td><td>Calories:</td></tr>
</table>

FATS	CARBS	PROTEINS	OTHERS

WATER □ □ □ □ □ □ □ □   ⏰ SLEEP   WEIGHT

WORKOUT ACTIVITIES / EXERCISES	SET / REPS / DISTANCE	CALORIES BURNED	TIME SPENT

NOTES/TODAY'S ACHIEVEMENT	WHAT WILL DO BETTER TOMORROW

M T W T F S S   MOOD   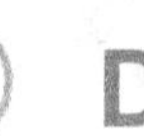   **DAY** 88

DATE ....

TODAY'S COMMITMENTS

____

____

____

TODAY MEALS	BREAKFAST	LUNCH	DINNER	SNACKS
	Calories:	Calories:	Calories:	Calories:

FATS	CARBS	PROTEINS	OTHERS

WATER ⏣ ⏣ ⏣ ⏣ ⏣ ⏣ ⏣ ⏣   SLEEP   WEIGHT

WORKOUT ACTIVITIES / EXERCISES	SET / REPS / DISTANCE	CALORIES BURNED	TIME SPENT

NOTES/TODAY'S ACHIEVEMENT	WHAT WILL DO BETTER TOMORROW

M T W T F S S   MOOD 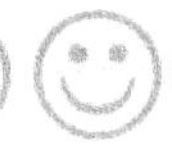  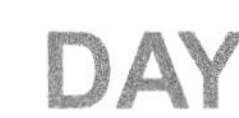   **DAY** | 89

DATE ....

TODAY'S COMMITMENTS

TODAY MEALS	BREAKFAST	LUNCH	DINNER	SNACKS
	Calories:	Calories:	Calories:	Calories:

FATS	CARBS	PROTEINS	OTHERS

WATER ⬜⬜⬜⬜⬜⬜⬜⬜   SLEEP   WEIGHT

WORKOUT ACTIVITIES / EXERCISES	SET / REPS / DISTANCE	CALORIES BURNED	TIME SPENT

NOTES/TODAY'S ACHIEVEMENT	WHAT WILL DO BETTER TOMORROW

M T W T F S S   MOOD   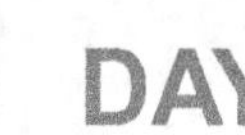   **DAY** 90

DATE ....

TODAY'S COMMITMENTS

TODAY MEALS	BREAKFAST	LUNCH	DINNER	SNACKS
Calories:	Calories:	Calories:	Calories:

FATS	CARBS	PROTEINS	OTHERS

WATER ☐ ☐ ☐ ☐ ☐ ☐ ☐ ☐   SLEEP   WEIGHT

WORKOUT ACTIVITIES / EXERCISES	SET / REPS / DISTANCE	CALORIES BURNED	TIME SPENT

NOTES/TODAY'S ACHIEVEMENT	WHAT WILL DO BETTER TOMORROW

90 Days Milestone Achievement Reward Chart...

MILESTONE	REWARDS

90 Days Milestone Achievement Reward Chart...

MILESTONE	REWARDS
MILESTONE	REWARDS

HELLO NEW ME!

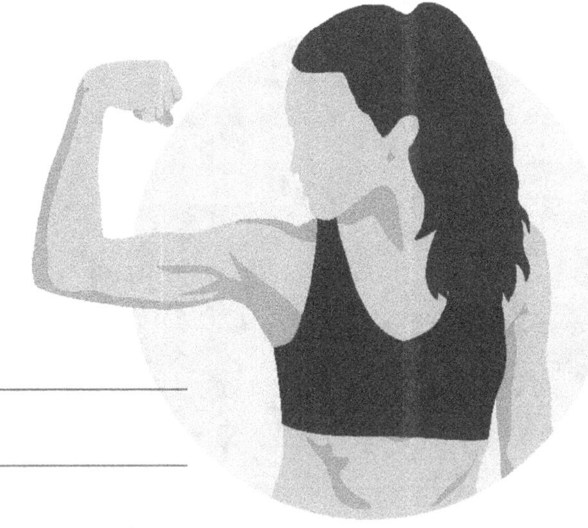

Neck _______________

Arm _______________

Chest _______________

Waist _______________

Hip _______________

Thigh _______________

Calf _______________

BMI _______________

Weight

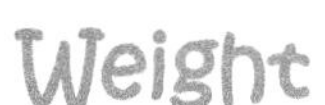

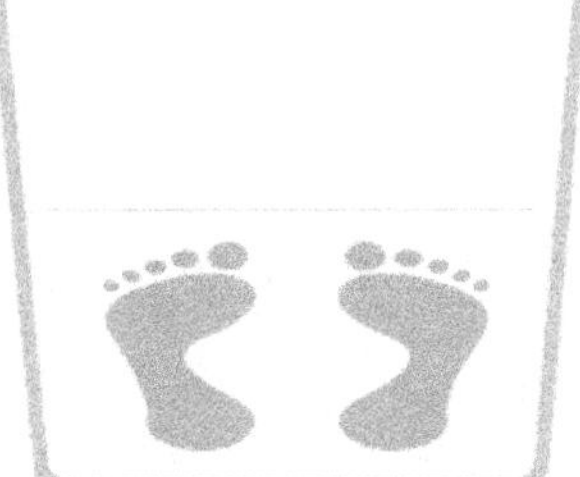

RESULTS _______________

____

____

____

____

Notes

www.ingramcontent.com/pod-product-compliance
Lightning Source LLC
Chambersburg PA
CBHW070746250726
48662CB00004B/1660